Gloriously Grateful

*A Journey Through the Diagnosis
and Treatment of Colon Cancer Told
with Compassion and Humor*

MARION ANDREWS

GLORIOUSLY GRATEFUL

A Journey Through the Diagnosis and
Treatment of Colon Cancer Told with
Compassion and Humor

Marion Andrews
1527 Hilton Parma Corners Road
Spencerport, NY 14559
(585) 495-2435

ISBN: 978-1-7342310-0-7

Design by Transcendent Publishing

Printed in the United States of America.

DEDICATION

This book is dedicated to both sides of the equation: the patient (without patience) and the caregiver (who needs the lion's share).

Additionally, this is dedicated to the special people who have come along on this great adventure and journey with me.

ACKNOWLEDGMENTS

First, to my husband, Dave. I am so deeply thankful that you are part of my life, and that you took such good care of me over those three years of seemingly endless doctors, scans, procedures, and treatments. My gratitude is forever.

I am also incredibly grateful to my sister Anne. Though we live thousands of miles apart, you have been with me every single day in love. Thank you.

To my daughter Michelle and her wife, Dani. Thank you for coming to be with me whenever you could, for your silent encouragement and, always, your love. You are a constant reminder of how to live with laughter, even on bad days.

To all those special loved ones who were there to drive me back and forth to the clinic and cheer me up with a word or a hug - thank you for hanging in with me.

CONTENTS

FOREWORD

I was so excited when I heard that Marion Andrews was writing a book about her journey with cancer, and deeply honored when she asked me to write the forward. Marion and I have had a special relationship for my entire life – literally. You see, Marion is not only my dear friend and co-author of the best-selling self-discovery guided journal, *Who Am I, Anyway?* She is also my mother. Since I was part of the journey, before and after cancer, it made perfect sense to share my perspective and how important it is for everyone to read *Gloriously Grateful.*

As I read through it for the first time, I understood so much more about what Mom went through and what she learned from her experiences. Though I had witnessed most of it firsthand, there were still many things I wasn't aware of, and now that I am, I'm even prouder of her for sharing her story with such openness.

My whole life, Mom, has been there for me, lending her support, intelligence, humor, and, most of all, love. Always very close, we grew even more so when I was diagnosed with Chronic Fatigue Syndrome (CFS) as a teenager. Mom discovered she had been living with CFS for the previous ten years, and my sickness triggered her to have a CFS relapse. Over the next several years, we spent even more time together, often just sitting for hours, giving each other strength and comfort.

As I grew into adulthood, my symptoms improved, and life led me in different directions. For many years I've lived two thousand miles away, and in between visits, we maintained our strong connection through text messages and regular video calls. Life was good, and as like most people, we did not think of, plan, or prepare for this type of situation, so when it happened, we were shaken to the core.

Mom's family comes from very strong stock. Her parents lived long and healthy lives filled with love and energy. She's the youngest of eight, and at the time of this writing, all her siblings are still alive. So it was shocking and surreal to find out that at just sixty-five years old, she would have to deal with such a severe and life-threatening condition.

Our journey was particularly challenging because I lived so far away and wasn't in a position to spend long periods of time with her. We are great at just being together and keeping each other company, and if I lived closer, I would've been able to help her at home and take her to chemo treatments and doctor visits. Not being able to do so was very difficult for both of us.

Throughout this journey, laughter has been our saving grace. Mom and I have always shared a sense of humor, finding ways to laugh no matter the struggle. I remember, even in the toughest times, the smallest things are the funniest, like the fact that I'm so uncoordinated that I trip easily and often run into walls. It can be quite amusing, just watching me walk! Of course, it is tricky to find things to laugh about when dealing with cancer, but we did what we could to find humor and healing where we could.

Our animal friends also played a role in this journey, providing much comfort and comic relief. I have always adored animals, especially cats, and in 2012 I adopted two adorable ones. First came Oscar Lee, a grey and white tabby who is not only the most loving cat I've ever owned but the one with the loudest purr. When I first got Oscar, he would cry at the door when I left for work and come running when I got home. To keep Oscar company, my tall, sleek black Java Bean joined the family. Oscar and Java immediately bonded and, if you didn't know any different, you would think they came from the same litter.

Mom loves spending time with Oscar and Java when she visits. Each has a strong, distinct personality and a natural love of entertaining. Oscar loves to hunt and play with the green lid stoppers we bring home from coffee shops. Java is a real talker and likes to "supervise" Mom's bathroom visits, telling her stories the entire time. He also enjoys cuddling up beside her while she sleeps!

When we couldn't be together, I helped Mom by sending her many, many photos of the cats with all their healing adorableness. I also recorded Oscar purring and randomly sent the audios to Mom so he could share his love too, as well as videos of the kitty antics, some of which were genuinely hilarious. Each time Mom gets one, I know I have brightened her day and that Oscar and Java are doing their part to help her heal. Oscar also likes to participate in our regular FaceTime chats.

Intellectually I knew she had cancer. Emotionally, I knew on some levels, but more often, it felt like it was a bad dream. There were a few things that brought the point home.

When Mom was going through her first round of chemo treatments, I visited her during her final chemo treatment. There she was, her head wrapped in scarf instead of her usual full hair, sitting in the chair with chemicals flowing into her system to destroy the cancer cells. It was extremely scary to see such a strong, seemingly indestructible person in this incredibly vulnerable situation. Suddenly the possibility of my losing her became very, very real.

At the same time, it was amazing to witness Mom's transformation during this time. She began exploring her creative side, which I found incredibly cool, having kept journals my entire life and dabbled with sketching and other crafts since I was a teen living with CFS.

Mom discovered the therapeutic joys of journaling, drawing, and letting her brain freely explore new things. It was fun and still is, to see the beautiful work she creates with her hand-drawn and stamped homemade all-occasion cards, and I was so glad to know that she wrote about this part of her journey in this book.

The honesty, humor, and heart Mom brings to *Gloriously Grateful* makes it a must-read for everyone whose lives have been touched, directly or indirectly, by cancer. Mom shares the ups and downs, insights, fears, and surprises that cancer brought and changed her life. You'll discover how important it is to listen to your body, stay persistent, and fight for what you know to be true about yourself. Even when something seemed like it could be ignored, Mom's refusal to stop asking questions saved her life. Most importantly, you will realize that you're not alone, whether you have been diagnosed with cancer or are going through it with someone you love.

Michelle Forsyth

CHAPTER ONE

The Journey Begins

*I*t began with some pain in my abdomen. At times, sharp pain. Distressing pain. Unfamiliar pain. I went to the doctor, who was unsure of the cause and ordered a series of trial and error tests, visits to specialists, and various medications. Nothing we tried worked. I continued to experience the pain plus a distinct feeling that my stomach was rolling and undulating. It was also making loud whooshing sounds like Niagara Falls. Then I began vomiting after eating. Now, this was highly unusual for me. I never throw up and will fight the feeling with total concentration. The only times in my life I threw up consistently were when I was pregnant with each of my three children. At nearly sixty-six years old, post-menopausal, and having had "the plumbing" removed fifteen years before, I was sure we could rule pregnancy out. Still, my stomach roared and trembled. Maybe an ulcer? I tried some new medications, and I restricted my foods to very bland choices. No, this did not help either. Nearly six months went by with these very unusual symptoms.

I kept going back to the doctor because I knew my own body and knew something was wrong. The lesson here is to trust yourself. Trust your feelings and keep going through the system until you are satisfied. Finally, my doctor ordered an endoscopy to have a look at my innards from the top down. The results were typical except for an unusual redness and irritation near my duodenum, the place where the stomach joins the intestines. He proposed a colonoscopy to check this out. What?? I'd had one two and a half years earlier and was given a clean slate—no polyps; nothing but clean, healthy intestines in there. I was opposed. I have seven siblings and hundreds of other relatives, I told him, and not one case of colon cancer among them. To my way of thinking, this was extremely low on the list of probable causes. He kept insisting that this was the next step in determining what was going on. Finally, I agreed, thinking it was going to be a complete waste of time.

The doctor scheduled the procedure for the next Friday, June 13, four days before my birthday. Nice birthday present! I had a friend drive me, and our conversation centered around where we would go for brunch after the test was over. I went in grumbling but resigned. The doctor was ready to start, but the nurse had not yet given me the injection that sent me to la-la land. I was able to watch the progress on the monitor. See! I knew it, nothing but a lovely pink, healthy colon. Then an ugly-looking sore showed up. EEEWWW.

What was that?

The doctor began snipping off little pieces. *That is nasty. Why is he doing that?* was my last thought as I slipped into that drugged sleep. The next thing I knew, I was waking up groggily, with my friend sitting next to the bed. I was anxious to get up and out of there and have some breakfast. After the days of preparation for this test, plus all the days of trial and error diet modifications, I just wanted to get to a restaurant and have some solid food and a cup of coffee. When the doctor came in to give me the report, he spoke softly and was serious. He proceeded to tell me that he found a sizable growth in my ascending colon and had taken tissue samples for testing. He also said that I needed a CT scan immediately. His nurse would be calling me that afternoon with the scheduled time for Monday. He had expedited the samples of the biopsy so we would get those back quickly. Still under the influence of the drugs, I did not understand the gist of what he was saying. With food on my mind, I kept smiling and thanking him profusely. Yes, yes, thank you.

I escaped as quickly as possible, and we made a beeline for the nearest restaurant. The cafe was only about ten minutes away, and we hurried in. I was drinking coffee and waiting for my meal when my cell phone rang. It was Dave, my husband, and he had a very urgent message for me. Our primary care doctor had called and left a message that I would most likely need surgery right away. Did I want him to begin the process of getting an appointment with a surgeon? My husband was entirely justified in the panic he was feeling. I assured him I would call back as soon as the office opened after lunch. No problem! This was a time of blissful ignorance.

I was still of the mindset that nothing serious could be wrong, given my family history, as well as my own. I had regular colonoscopies that were always clean and clear. I ate an abundance of grains and wholesome food, had never smoked, and drank plenty of water. In short, I was the one who always tried to take good care of my health. All the fuss about CT scans and surgery just was not making it through my drugged mind at that point.

The reality hit me a few hours later when I talked with our doctor. The gastroenterologist had called him with his findings, and they were both quite sure this was critical. Shock and dismay! What was this all about? I asked the one question that I did not want to have him answer: could this be cancer? He was very considerate and honest in his answer. There was an extremely high possibility that this was colon cancer, though he would not say for sure until they had the report of the biopsies taken earlier during the test.

Whoa! That news hit me like a ton of bricks. It is hard to describe the emotions that surged through my body from head to toe; I can say shock and terror were fighting for the lead. The terror came in part because our doctor was fast-tracking everything; in fact, I already had an appointment with the surgeon the next Wednesday.

At this point, I did not tell many people. I was keeping this close to my chest in the hopes that it was all a mistake. Dave and I walked into the surgeon's office that day with a great deal of anticipation and dread. The surgeon was straightforward and kind. After telling us that the reports of the biopsy samples from the colonoscopy were not back yet, he went on to discuss possible scenarios and answer our "what-if" questions. I appreciated his candor. I am the kind of person who likes the facts and information laid out. I need to know what is what, and then I can deal with it.

At this point, I was also trying to keep things low key for my husband. He can be much more affected than I am, so some of my attention was on getting the information as quickly as possible and facing this head-on so he would not feel panicked. Plus concentrating on him and his reaction kept me from thinking about what was going on in my gut. As we were about to leave, the surgeon decided to check once more to see if the office had received the results. Yes, the report was there. Yes, it was a tumor about four centimeters wide, and it was malignant. The word "malignant," ouch "cancer," hit me – whoosh! - like an eighteen-wheeler, and I realized how hard I had been clinging to hope. Scarcely able to breathe, I had no idea what Dave was feeling or how he was reacting. My focus was now on me! I needed to escape. We left as quickly as possible.

The staff scheduled the surgery within a week. Oh my! Everything was in motion, and I was stunned as if I had entered an alternate reality. I was going on with the ordinary things of life, making meals, shopping, talking to friends, and yet the central part of my brain was grappling with that big C word – CANCER. And then the words "colon cancer" would flash across that brain screen. The people I'd heard of who had colon cancer were no longer alive. The prospect that I could die crossed my mind.

At this point, I knew I needed to calm down and get in touch with my inner self. Get centered and grounded. It had been many years since I consciously thought of these concepts. When I was much younger, I spent uncountable hours reading and listening to many motivational speakers. I believed without a doubt that "thoughts are things," and they could shape my future. These ideas had been put on the back burner for the past 20 years of divorces and marriages, moving from place to place, and one big move from Canada to the USA. I had been drifting along, more or less mindlessly. Of course, I was involved in many activities, "busy work" volunteering, and always in a learning mode intellectually and socially but mostly ignoring my spiritual needs. In this time of crisis, this came flooding back to me. I realized that I needed to spend time in contemplation and prayer. When I connected inwardly, the message I heard was that this was a time of change. I needed to allow my inner strength and determination to get me through this ordeal. I have always been a very spiritual person, not so much religious, with a firm belief and knowledge that my real being is a spirit housed in a physical body. I had searched for my purpose here on earth my whole life. It seemed to me that since I was not sure of my mission, I might still have work to do. The first job was to deal with this disease. I did not have any idea of what the result of this would be, but I was going to face it as best as I could. I can assure you that I was *not* feeling grateful for anything that was happening right at this time. Two things came to my rescue. One, I am a positive person, and that was sustaining me in the background. Two, I am always examining things that happen to me with the intention of searching out the lesson I am to learn from the situation. Now it appears that I had a whole lot of learning to do.

As my mind settled down, I was better able to see the steps before me. Now that surgery was scheduled, I needed to tell my family and friends, but how? Where would I start? How do I tell them? I knew I needed to be open and forthright. Doing this "telling" in person would be the most desirable, but since I happen to live thousands of miles from my family, that was not an option.

Thus began a flurry of calls and emails. The hardest thing was breaking the news to my children. There was lots of emotion on that call, but we got through it. I assured them that no one needed to come flying out as it was not that kind of emergency. Yes, I would have loved to have all three of them and their families close at hand, but I knew that it was not possible. Next, I called the sister with whom I have the closest relationship and, as calmly as possible, explained the plan for the surgery and more biopsies. These results would help determine the types of treatment we could face. She, too, was understandably tearful and frightened for me.

I then relayed the news to my other siblings, while my husband phoned his children and did the same. I also called or emailed my closest friends. Why? It was not to elicit sympathy or pity, but because I knew that I would need many positive, supportive people around me to deal with this. I am usually a very private person, putting on a brave face, dealing with everyone's issues and illnesses. Somehow, instinctively, I knew that this was NOT a time for that. I knew that I would need and want as much help, prayer, and support that I could muster.

CHAPTER TWO

New List

~ 🦋 ~

 efore I knew it the day of the surgery had arrived. My attitude: let's get on with it and move on to the next step. A piece of cake, right? Turns out, not so much. They removed ten to twelve inches of my ascending colon and nineteen lymph nodes that looked suspicious. The doctor said the surgery went well. I wasn't sure exactly what that meant, though I presumed it was that he was able to remove the "bad parts" of my colon and the offending lymph nodes and stitch everything back together. Now, from my perspective, it wasn't an apparent success. My insides refused to come back online. This little snag initiated an hourly check from a nurse. They so patiently came in, listened to my lower abdomen for life signs, rumbling, grumbling, anything! The irony did not escape my notice. Before surgery, my insides sounded like Niagara Falls on an angry day. Now, after a snip and trim, nothing! I could not eat until we had lower bowel noises, so water and ice chips were the delicious menus of each day. They had to put a tube down my nose to drain my stomach and keep it empty of gastric juices. Here is when the Universe/God and His angels took care of me.

At this time, I had not studied angels or any of the heavenly helpers. Sure, I knew the basic things from childhood, but my adult learning was sadly limited. Yet, the angels were watching over me. I had had just one Reiki treatment a month before this discovery. The woman, who later became my friend and Reiki Master, lived close to the hospital, told me she felt she needed to come up to see me. That day, she sat beside me with her hands on my abdomen and poured Reiki, which is unique energy from God and the Universe, into my body. I began to feel better, and within a few hours, the steady flow of energy got things realigned and moving. My faith in a Universal God and other heavenly creatures was there in the distance. The subconscious mind remembers, and these recent events triggered my response. I did not know that soon I was going to learn a whole lot more about Reiki and the energy that is available to us if we ask. I was going to use and work with this reawakened faith. In a few more days, the medical staff discharged me from the hospital.

The month of July was a blur of activity. I heard about treatment possibilities, including chemotherapy and all its side effects, as well as radiation. In the cancer clinic's doctor's opinion, radiation was less desirable because there was more than one cancer site. This whole exercise was incredibly complicated and often confusing. I listened, trying to understand what would be involved. There seem to be so many decisions to be made around all the various available treatments.

I had said long ago that if I ever had cancer, I would *not* have chemotherapy. Putting that poison into my body to kill the cancer cells and, by the way, a lot of the healthy cells ("collateral damage" is the term), was *not* something I wanted to do *ever*! But and it's a big *but*, when the time comes to face this front and center, things look a little different. When I heard the odds of surviving Stage 3B colon cancer (meaning it had already metastasized to some lymph nodes) with and without chemo, the choice was obvious. Without treatment, I had an eighty percent chance of dying within a year. With treatment, those odds went down to a twenty percent chance of dying. Or, a better way to look at it was that with treatments, I had an eighty percent chance of outliving this creature called cancer. I would take the chemo.

Next then, was to get set up with an oncologist and learn more about the therapy. The recommended plan was a combination of drugs to be administered every two weeks for six months. I had a tour of the clinic, was shown where to check in for the blood tests, and where the actual treatment would happen. It was all like being on a merry-go-round: a whirlwind tour, with just glimpses of what was to come. I hadn't yet pic-tured myself in one of those chairs with an IV pole beside me. It was like watching a movie; I was a spectator, and all the doctors, physician assistants, nurses, technicians, volunteers with coffee and treats were the cast of players. I continued in this observant role when telling my family and friends about the cancer and the treatment schedule. These scenes of a play were happening, but it seemed not to *me*.

Then a new wrinkle appeared. Before beginning chemo, my every bodily function had to be monitored and baselines recorded so they could administer the treatment as safely as possible, with minimal risk of complications. The many tests included a cardiological assessment, as I would be getting a port in my upper chest to accommodate the infusion needle, with a tube leading directly to my heart. It became apparent during these tests that I needed an electrocardiogram because I had "funny" wiring in my heart. Was this another potentially life-threatening condition? I was relieved to find out that it was "normal" for me, a bundle branch anomaly that had been there for many years and not a cause of concern. Still, it was one more thing I had to deal with, besides coming to terms with the diagnosis, the insertion of the port, and the treatment itself. Each one of these steps required an immense amount of energy, faith, and resolve.

The treatments were scheduled to begin August 1, 2014, which coincidentally is my daughter's birthday. It was a memorable day in so many ways, and I could now add this adventure to that list.

As we headed to the cancer clinic for my first infusion, I tried to think of how happy I was on that day decades earlier, when that beautiful baby girl joined our family. It brought me a little glimmer of joy and gratitude in an otherwise terrifying day. Sure, I had that visitor's tour of the clinic when getting set up. But that was the scenic tour – this was the real deal! It was all business now. Again, this smacked me right in the face. I was here at the clinic for treatment, which, OMG, meant that, yes, I for sure did have that nasty C-word. It was bizarre.

I have always been an optimistic, sunshiny-day kind of person, but handling the cancer clinic experience took all my energy and every bit of grit that I had. First, they put the injection needle in the port to be ready to infuse the drugs and take the blood samples they need to test before you begin. The required needle insertion happened in a completely sterile environment, right down to my wearing a mask and turning my head away from the site until it is covered and sealed. The line would go directly into a catheter that threads into a large vein above the right side of the heart called the superior vena cava, so they were super careful that no germs or bacteria were allowed in. Still, if I was feeling shaky before, pure old fear now presented its ugly head. I was terrified.

Again, the mantra "Thoughts are things" reverberated through my mind, and I realized I needed to be as careful with my thoughts as the doctors were with this line, protecting my virtual heart from any "germs" just as they were protecting my physical one. I was, and still am, so thankful for all the seminars and weekend conferences I had attended, learning from some of the best thinkers about positive input. There were also the incredible books I had read, like *The Power of Positive Thinking* by Norman Vincent Peale; *Think and Grow Rich* by Napoleon Hill; and Maxwell Maltz's 1960 classic *Psycho-Cybernetics*. Talks by motivational and self-help gurus Zig Ziglar, Charles Nelson Reilly, Brian Tracey, and more flooded my mind with the sure knowledge that the way we think directly impacts who we are and our health. In more recent years, I have learned from other great thinkers, including Louise Hay, Oprah Winfrey, Dr. Wayne Dyer, and Dr. Joe Dispenza. If these are unfamiliar to you, I suggest you investigate one or two of them.

Psycho-Cybernetics, in particular, blew my mind and would be my first recommendation to others. One of the analogies Maltz uses is how we learn to drive a car. Remember that at first, you needed to mentally rehearse all the steps before you put the car in gear. Later, as you became familiar with the routine, you just jumped in, started it, and took off. Boom! Through repetition, we have conditioned our minds to change a difficult task into a rote one, with no specific thought needed. Logically, if repetition works for this type of task, we can also use it to train ourselves to think and respond positively to outside stimuli automatically.

All it takes is repetition or practice. I needed every bit of positive reinforcement to get through the next months.

When I was reading and learning from these brilliant works, I did not know that I was preparing my mind and spirit for the battle with this disease. It is interesting to me that I was on a path, working with and for my purpose here on earth, even when I didn't understand what that was or realize that it was happening for me and my future.

One of the things I am most grateful for is that this cancer, treatment, and recovery has finally made me understand and feel one hundred percent assured of my purpose here on earth. Before this adventure, I thought I had no clear idea of what I was to do "down here"; it was the question I asked most often when in discussion with some of the wisest people I knew. Why am I here? What is my purpose? Really, what am I supposed to be doing here? I believe in a God/Higher Power who is infinitely wise, and in my humble opinion, would not send souls to earth in a willy-nilly fashion with no purpose or plan. I believe that we have the blueprint of this plan embedded in our subconscious minds, and we need to figure that out and accomplish some, if not all, of that plan during our lifetime here on earth.

Now it was time to dig out all those positive ideas, learnings, and techniques I had jammed into my brain, heart, and soul. They would make it easier to deal with the weight of this – the fear, pain, and side effects – and help make the necessary decisions.

Of course, one of those decisions was whether to have the chemo and once I made it, I had very few second thoughts. It was as if the spiritual part of me said, *Yes, Yes! This treatment is what is needed right now.* I knew deep within my soul that this was my path to walk, that I needed to do this as a part of completing my life purpose. I realized I was here on earth to heal and to teach, and right now, I was being presented with the gift of walking in this disease so I could share my journey with others and help them heal, even as I helped myself. I was, and remain, humbled and grateful.

Then my other side, the ego, chimed in, "Hey, you! Is this necessary?" In the few weeks between the oncologist's discussion of treatments and the start date, many thoughts poured in. Scary thoughts. Nervous thoughts. Overwhelming thoughts. This was a whole new world I was entering. I was surprised that it was going to be six months of chemotherapy. I was sad, and often found myself asking, *Is this real?* I was also worried about Dave's reaction and how he was coping with all that was happening.

The next part of my mental preparation was just plain tough. The suggestions that the books and cancer-help websites offered were to visualize a final positive result. In my mind, I needed to live as a healthy, cancer-free person. I needed to expect this outcome. Then the thought, *But what if the results are not so pretty?* would pop up. I believe that the results do not matter as much as the journey – the learning that happens as we make the decisions and carry them out. In today's instantaneous world, we seem to have forgotten about the joy of the journey. We get information immediately, as it is happening. We turn on our computer, tablet, or smartphone and see our family or friends. Whatever is happening in any far-off land is promptly at our fingertips. Our impatience knows no bounds. We want it now! Remember when travel was fun? When a trip on an airplane was a great adventure? Now it's, "Are we there yet?" The cancer diagnosis and the treatments that followed – not to mention the subsequent return of the disease a few more times – reminded me of the need for patience and trying to capture the joy of the journey.

We all have many decisions and opportunities for learning along our individual journeys, even when something like cancer appears to rob us of all control. Decisions like trying to eat correctly. Choices of how we are going to approach each day. Happiness, joy, and gratitude are conscious decisions, just like learning how to drive. When we practice the routine repetitiously, these attributes will become part of us. None of this is easy. All of it is doable, and no matter what the results are, the journey is so worth it. But *OMG*, the road is something else.

The treatments were unbelievably hard on me, not only physically but mentally as well. I know the chemo drugs are powerful and, potentially, deadly. They kill the cancer cells but also do irreparable damage to healthy cells. So, each time I went to the clinic, I put myself in the position of having poison injected directly into my heart. I had to trust that the medical professionals had the dosage right. What a balancing act. Enough to kill the fast-growing cancer cells yet carefully still stopping short of killing the patient. Actually, the first few treatments were reasonably simple to handle. As I said, I had made the decision to go ahead with the treatments, so I did just that.

After a few months, I had to work at psyching myself up to go there. My treatments were booked for every other Friday. After each treatment, I would spend the first week too weak and physically sick to think about the next one. That week became an hour by hour of sheer willpower to stay alive. Sometimes every cell in my body protested. The desire to just give in and vegetate was overwhelming. Yet I knew I could not. This resolve was strengthened by a discipline that I didn't think I had. I used every tool that had been recommended to me. I learned to meditate, and I began a journal to write thoughts and feelings. I did self-Reiki treatments, plus went to my Reiki Master to administer them to me. Of course, I slept a great deal of the time. I prayed. I used a visualization technique that was suggested to me by a wise woman working with the archangels.

All these techniques and ideas had the welcome effect of also soothing my harried mind. I spent as much time as possible, though sometimes only minutes, in the comforting presence of the angels. These magnificent spirits are sent to help us, and allowing them into my life was a blessing like none other. I will always be grateful for the motivation that I found to begin to study and work with the many angels that God/Source has provided as helpers for us. I learned that because we have free will, we need to invite and invoke them in. Being so physically depleted made me finally receptive to getting to know these extraordinary beings. You can always be sustained by their loving presence, and especially when you are at your lowest point physically.

I have always believed that God/Source made us with a powerful mind and spirit and that it's our responsibility to use these gifts to figure out what we are to do with our lives. When I was at the point of almost total depletion from the disease and treatments, I was hit with the absolute realization that I was not alone in this inner battle but had many friends and loved ones willing to help. I had angels and archangels waiting and ready to support me as well. I had hundreds of people praying for whatever outcome was in my best interest.

CHAPTER THREE

Round One

Of course, there were many preparations I had to make before going to the clinic that first big day. What to take and wear were big decisions. I bought some comfortable knit pants and zip-up hoodies to wear. Keeping in mind that the port had to be accessible, I found some tank tops with scoop necks to accommodate this. I am usually hot and tend to wear light clothes. However, the stress and unknowns of this adventure, plus the general feeling of malaise, often made me feel very chilly. Warm socks and comfy slippers were necessary. The slippers with rubber soles were indispensable for taking my IV Pole buddy on excursions around the hallways. I packed a book, crafting supplies to make cards, put music on my phone, and grabbed my earphones. The social worker at the cancer clinic recommended journaling as a great tool, so some new blank journals went into my bag and, of course, new colorful pens. I am somewhat a collector of pens and markers, so this was a big choice. Nerd Alert! There is something very thrilling about opening a new, blank journal and choosing just the right pen to write those first words. Before getting to the actual writing, I would write my name and contact information on the inside cover. Seeing my name written there was exciting for me. This journal was now *my* book! *My* thoughts and ideas were going to be written in here. Sometimes I would write a motivational quote there as well. It was always such a joy to begin and still is. I warned you! I am a nerd and happy to be one.

Taking that trip to a stationery store (or even an online one) to buy a new journal was incredibly uplifting. Choosing a journal is a complicated task. First, I look at the fascinating and inviting array of covers of all the journals available. And there are a ton. There are serious ones made of leather, some simple but oh-so-luxuriously rich-looking and somber, while others are more lighthearted and fun, decorated with coffee cups, cookies, and other whimsical elements. Then there are the beautiful nature scenes that catch my eye (I love lakes, oceans, and mountain views), and those with gorgeous flowers on one side. For that first journal, I finally chose one that was pearlized with embossed butterflies. Isn't it glorious, I told myself, to have such a variety to choose from? I found a pretty pen that felt good in my hand. The nib was fine, and the ink flowed smoothly on the paper. Now I was ready!

Are you thinking? *What? All this effort to get a notebook and pen?* Yes, and I thoroughly enjoy this. There are many hard and unpleasant things to come in the next six months of treatments. I am grateful to have this tactile, physical pleasure of picking out a journal and pen, then holding it in my hands, and writing in it. Don't miss out on the ordinary, simple joys in this process—find a little sunshine wherever you can on a sometimes very dark and dreary journey.

Was I stressed through all of this? Well, a few days before my first treatment, I needed to get that electrocardiogram as a baseline and a precaution. I left the house, drove three or four miles, and realized that I had forgotten to put my partial plate of front teeth in. Whoops! I had a feeling as I was leaving the house that I was forgetting something. I checked for money and my phone, and both were there; I was good to go. As I was driving down the street, I ran my tongue over my gums, oh no! No front teeth! U-turn! Dash back to the house, grab them, in they go, then back on the road. It's always an adventure.

Now, let's look at the schedule of an infusion day at the clinic. First, there were blood tests to make sure I was okay to have the drugs. Words like "platelet counts" and "creatinine" now became part of my vocabulary. The next step was to meet with the oncologist to verify that it was a "go." Then back to the clinical wing for the actual infusion. It takes between four and five hours for this part of the treatment. Once these drugs are in your body, they put on a portable pump with the vials of drugs for the next forty-eight hours. After the nurse checked this out, I could go home, but the machine would stay on from Friday afternoon until Sunday afternoon, pumping in the rest of the drugs in the "cocktail." A home care nurse would then come and take it off; then, I was free for nearly two weeks.

And, oh yes, the pump was in an ever-stylish, oh-so-fashionable black fanny pack. Another first for me! I never owned or thought of having or wearing a fanny pack. And BONUS! No showering while wearing this modern fashion accessory. And all I wanted to do was shower to freshen up after a day at the cancer clinic—another thing to get used to with this regimen.

Along with the chemotherapy drugs, I have antinausea meds to take as well. I wonder, *Are these going to be necessary?* And at first, I am reluctant to add these to the stream of medication already in my body. But, oh yes, by Sunday, my system is rebelling, and the feeling of nausea is overwhelming. I HATE TO THROW UP!!! I fight it with every fiber of my being, but the gag reflex wins. Okay, okay, I'll take the drugs. This was one of those times when I was feeling defeated. Nausea came on like waves, and I am powerless to fight, and before I know it, I am in the bathroom. *Ohhh, I really, really hate this;* my mind is whirling. Now the choice is clear: take the &%**# drugs or spend the next few days hugging the white monster. No brainer. It is not worth the aggravation and the chance of getting even more rundown because I'm not getting any nutrition into my body. Once the nausea passed, I began to feel better, but not nearly close to "myself," as the before me. Chemo made me feel tired and ill for the next ten days. All told, I have three to four days of reasonably ordinary living before I had to go do this all over again.

Then there are the racing thoughts and questions that pop in and out of my mind as I sit in the clinic for the six hours of the infusion. Questions like, *When did this tumor start? I had that colonoscopy two and a half years ago, and it was perfect! Clear and clean. So, what's with this now?* I feel like I had been living my life the best I could and then – BOOM! – cancer is spreading in me and multiplying quickly. What happened to make it show up now? My Reiki Master suggested that the Reiki energy session I'd had back in May could have pulled the Universal Force toward me to make this show up so I could get treated and learn whatever lessons I needed to learn. Well, that was a bit woo-woo for me right now, but I tucked that idea away to consider later. These questions don't feel like "Why Me?" but rather, "Where the heck did this come from?" What stresses do I need to let go of to heal and stay healthy? I am ready and willing to change anything right now to heal and move on with my life.

Here's another thing: the cancer itself didn't hurt. There was no localized sharp pain at the actual place where they found the tumor. The pain that I felt in my abdomen was from the blockage, not directly from the cancer — the tumor blocking the colon was causing many confusing symptoms. I am so grateful for this small mercy. Many cancers are extremely painful, and eventually, this one would have been if left untreated. As mentioned, I had been diagnosed with Stage 3B colon cancer, which means that the cancer had moved out of the tumor to penetrate the colon walls. It gets a new title – Stage 4 – when the disease shows up in other areas. Stage 5 is unbelievably severe, so we don't want to go there. If I let my mind wander down that spiraling path, it is overwhelming. I say to myself. *It's only numbers and letters. I am strong and healthy. This place is not where my thoughts need to be.* I often have to catch myself, and consciously and forcefully make my thoughts return to positive things. Yes, sometimes, I didn't want to be optimistic anymore. I would then allow myself five or ten minutes to wallow and be miserable, then shut that off.

As you've gathered by now, the first day of infusion was no walk in the park! It was tiring, mentally exhausting, disheartening, and in some ways, a terrifying experience. Seeing all the others – including some teens – getting their chemo treatments was very hard. I was so grateful that I was older and had lived such a full and enjoyable life, yet there I was with all the other cancer patients. At that moment, my mind did not want to grasp this reality. It seemed this must be happening to someone else, and I was merely looking on from a distance. Because, because, there is no way that I could be the one with cancer. But the sad truth of it was the chemo drugs were flowing through that port, impossible to ignore. My friends picked me up after the day of treatment and took me home.

I wasn't sure why, but when getting these treatments, I wanted a ride to and from the clinic, then be left alone to muddle through the day. Others had family and friends with them in their treatment space. I did not. I wanted to, needed to, handle this part by myself. I have thought about this often. Later, during the next round, a friend would insist on being with me. But during those first six months of treatments, I just wanted to spend the time alone. I was not really alone, though. I was getting acquainted with my new self. I was vulnerable. I was sad. And yes, I was happy as well. I firmly believed that I was not the same person I had been just a few months earlier – pre-cancer. I wanted to beat this and explore the new me, post-cancer. I was not afraid of dying. I have never been. I had always looked forward to that new and exciting life "beyond the veil," as some call it. I was just not sure I was ready to go there right now.

The more time I spent in contemplation and meditation, the more I came to believe that I still had work to do in this world. That God/He/She/Spirit was not yet finished with me in this temporal body. The real essence of who I am is the spirit/soul – that was the true me. This outside physical self was merely handy for getting around this planet. I was grateful for this information. As I sat and listened to soft music, it was like the Universe was downloading all sorts of ideas into my brain. I was at peace spiritually. Physically, my body was being ravaged by the drugs that are killing the cancer cells.

I visualized the destroying of the cancer as much as I could, seeing the chemo almost like PacMan, eating all the bad cancer cells. (Google that game if you are too young to remember it.) Munch, munch, chomp, chomp. Perhaps this seems silly right now, but at that point, I was willing to do anything recommended to get that cancer out of my body. Visualization was part of it. There was always a glimmer of hope within me. Sure, it was dim on some days and bright on others, but I clung to that little light. In my mind and spirit, I wanted to make it through this, even when my body seemed ready to throw in the towel. It takes one small step forward to get to the end. It is necessary to make those baby steps every day.

CHAPTER FOUR

Extra Surprises

*O*ne of the most well-known and obvious side effects of chemo is hair loss. The staff told me that this particular drug cocktail might not cause my hair to fall out at all. So, while in a wait-and-see mode, I discussed this with other cancer survivors and patients. I also spent a lot of time thinking about it and told myself, "It's no big deal. I don't care that much; it's only hair and will grow back." BUT, as with most things that we try to prepare for and think we have settled in our minds, a surprise was imminent. Soon, every time I ran my hand through my hair, it came away with lots of loose strands. And I didn't like it! I really didn't like it! In fact, it brought up many feelings that are new and scary. What a revelation! Like the choice of having chemo or not, this is another time when I discovered that you couldn't know how you will feel about something until you are at that point. I had always taken my hair more or less for granted. It was thick and easy to deal with my whole life. Just shampoo, blow-dry, and I was done. Maybe that's why dealing with this loss is so much harder than I thought it would be. Wait-and-see mode over, I was off to my dear friend and hairdresser for a short, short cut – an interim until it all fell out.

Here is how I expressed this time in my journal:

This hair thing has me trying hard to get my sunny outlook back. It will come, but just for tonight, I think I am giving myself permission to grieve a little, pout a little, maybe shed a tear or two. Just a short detour, but it will be okay! I will be back on track, one foot in front of the other, a cheery smile on my face. I have an appointment coming up with a hairdresser who specializes in wigs and scarves and hats for those of us who lose their hair either through disease or chemo. I don't know what I will choose from her selection, maybe only scarves and hats, perhaps a wig. I really and truly don't know.

Maybe I am done with the pouting and nearly perhaps done with the grief over my hair loss. There are so many different emotions around this whole cancer thing that it is hard for others to understand. Sometimes I think that I am finished with the grieving and am moving forward and then – oh-oh! – it comes back and over some different part of this journey, onto the next day.

There are some fascinating experiences with my short new brush cut and steadily thinning hair. One day I was out when a rain cloud burst. Huge big raindrops were coming down, and for the first time in my life, I felt these big drops hitting my head!! Splash, splash. I don't think they even touched my hair.

Boomers on my scalp! These hurt. I would never have imagined that rain would hurt my head. How do bald men handle that all the time? I guess I needed to wear a hat or one of the cute bonnets I bought the previous week. In time, I would come to love the daily adventures that this disease and treatment brought to me.

Another exciting time was when I was driving along the road, enjoying the gorgeous warm day. I rolled down the windows instead of using the AC. Anyone who knows me knows how I hate the wind blowing my hair around. It truly gives me a headache when that happens. HEY! I found out that hair that is less than an inch long doesn't blow around! Hallelujah! The wind just whistled through my shorn locks and felt so refreshing. May have even whisked away any dandruff that was there! BONUS. Joyful day! Life is good.

Hair loss has another effect that I didn't expect: it made me, perhaps for the first time, genuinely feel like a cancer patient. The new wig did it, so did the bonnets. Am I really in chemotherapy???? Yes, it was still hard to get my head around that, and I found I needed to put off this idea a bit longer. Maybe I would deal with it tomorrow. Tonight, I would hit the wall at about six p.m. – not much moving around after that. Rest is required to deal with this continuous roller coaster ride.

Each chemo cycle has been different. Some were

not too bad physically, with only waves of yucky feelings. Tiredness would remain a significant hurdle throughout. If I was active, out with friends, for a few hours, I knew I would pay for it later! It was not so much sleepy tired as it was bone-weary exhaustion when even something like typing a short note is too much. It takes two hands to raise a cup of tea to my lips. It's times like this when your partner or support team needs to be very understanding and even more supportive. This is a time when friends and family are a great comfort with words, cards, and just the loving feelings they generate. This fight was more challenging than I ever could have imagined. I was so grateful for the people in my life, even those who offered love and support from a distance. A note for those in the caregiver role: sometimes, all you need to do is be there. No judgment, no expectations; just love, and your presence (be it in person, over the phone, or even email) is enough.

The next treatment was uneventful. I had my port draw almost immediately and then grabbed a mocha coffee while waiting for the results. My platelet count was good; kidney function was okay too, so it's full speed ahead. While I was sitting there getting the first two meds infused, I anticipated going home early, for a nap, my ever-stylish fanny pack pump strapped to me. I am feeling quite good today. The tiredness has passed for now, and I think it was likely due in part to the anticipation of today's treatment. I am sitting in a comfortable chair, with a heated blanket, listening to Pandora Radio, and typing in my journal at caringbridge.org. This is a free site set up, especially for cancer patients. I created an online journal to keep friends and family updated on my continuing journey battling colon cancer.

I'd had some good days, some terrible days, and then – surprise! – I had a great one. The sun was shining; it was not hot, but a glorious fall day. Just right! And I felt great! I spent the morning on errands, and with a nap after lunch, I was energized for the rest of the day. My biggest problem to date was fatigue, but with enough naps, I was getting through.

The wigs were a whole different experience. One, in particular, seemed to have a life of its own. It would start out feeling good and right, and then I would sense this movement of something sliding up on my head. It was subtle and slow, but it kept creeping until … Well, let me tell you a story the day I went to the clinic for treatment #4.

I thought I looked so good that day: wig hair on and makeup just right – I even used eye shadow. After an hour or so, I made a trip to the bathroom. I looked in the mirror, and wow, there was a peak of wig-hair poking up on the top of my head! And with the creeping wig, my hairline was showing, along with the cute under cap that looks like the hairnet of the cleaning lady or the cafeteria worker on *The Carol*

Burnett Show. Well, I pulled that wig back in place and then kept tugging at the temple pieces for the rest of the afternoon. If I had brought a hat or bonnet, I would have ripped the wig off altogether and stuffed it in my bag. But I didn't, so I was stuck doing wig maintenance all afternoon.

The next week meant a trip out to the salon where I bought that wig so the woman could adjust it. The last thing I needed was my hair flying off my head in the middle of the grocery store! I also bought an adorable hat at the salon – adorable except for its color: PINK. Now, I am sooo NOT a hat person and even less a pink person. For those who haven't known me my whole life, I have NEVER owned anything pink, nor did I dress my daughter in pink when she was a baby. Don't ask why because I don't know, but I have never liked pink on or near me. It's a beautiful color on others, just not me. Yet there I was with – I had to admit – a rather endearing pink hat, the only one in the salon that looked half decent on me. This journey was certainly turning into a life-rearranging experience. I would come to realize I do like pink, and I *loved* this new hat.

Another thing I learned was I am creative – almost artistic, even. One of the clinic's suggestions was to find some avenue to do something fun and exciting with your hands. I am a computer person. I can and do create beautiful cards and other types of artistic banners and posters on my computer. Yet now I found myself creating cards from scratch using various papers, stamping materials, and embellishments – a hobby I found both relaxing and intriguing. Who knew? Enforced rest and limited energy bring you to different doors. Playing with paper and ink was another new experience and one I was thoroughly enjoying.

In the working world, Wednesday has always been known as "hump day," meaning we are that much closer to the weekend. For me, hump day of every other week meant I was that much closer to my next treatment. On the Wednesday before treatment #5, something worrisome cropped up: I had a cough, and it was getting a bit bothersome. If it were still hanging on the next day, I would have to call the cancer center to see what I should do. With a compromised immune system, a cough can be a danger sign. I would talk to the experts and see if it needed to be checked out. Otherwise, this cycle had been good, with only a few stomach protests that were easily controlled with an antidiarrhea medication.

Every once in a while, I would be hit by a wave of anger. *Why, and what's the deal!* This disease was so unexpected – I had never even considered the possibility. Yes, I do like to control things in my life, and my health was one of the things I felt that I had under control. After years of dealing with fibromyalgia and Chronic Fatigue Syndrome (CFS), I had taken care to monitor my energy, budget my time, and observe all areas of my health with regular checkups and careful planning. But this just hit out of the blue! I worked at getting by the anger because I knew it served no purpose in my healing and promoted negative energy. I know some will say a bit of anger is a good thing. Anger may motivate some people, but it usually just makes me sad. I need positive motivation and positive input, and during that time, I worked exceptionally hard to maintain that attitude.

Music had always been an important part of my life, and I would find it a lifesaver now. I love music of almost any genre. I have a collection of songs from the 1940s and the latest in soft rock and new country. During my journey, many lyrics would pop into my head like unexpected little treats. Just a few words of a chorus that I sang along to with my sisters, or a rock-and-roll tune from Melissa Ethridge or Billy Joel as I drove along a highway, would take me on a short fun trip, out of the ugly present and into a different time and place.

One song that was popular on the country channel at this time was Dierks Bentley's "I Hold On." It spoke directly to what I was doing... holding on. The next line talks about holding on to things we count on to keep going strong. Also valid for me. I had experienced those dreaded symptoms yesterday, and though I felt normal today, tomorrow would be another treatment. I wanted to get there and be done, yet I dreaded this lethargic feeling and annoying diarrhea that hit so often. On the bright side, I was not feeling nauseous and had only minimal burning sensations in my hands and feet. I had a sensitivity to cold in my outer limbs, which I would often forget until I stuck my hand in the freezer to grab some food. Yikes! I would have to stop and grab a hot potholder to get that done. Minor irritations. Get on with it! Let go of the past and enjoy TODAY. Yes, I will, because I HOLD ON.

CHAPTER FIVE

Oh, Oh Oxaliplatin

*P*art of the chemo cocktail is a drug called Oxaliplatin. This drug can cause some unpleasant side effects, so it is monitored carefully. This drug can cause a reaction around treatment five or six. Usual side effects are peripheral neuropathy – numbness and tingling and cramping of the hands or feet often triggered by cold, mouth sores, and fatigue. I experienced all of these during those first few months of treatment. The feeling of difficulty swallowing, shortness of breath, jaw spasms, abnormal tongue sensation, and chest pressure are rare but possible occurrences. About one hour into the infusion on treatment #5, I started to feel very hot, very sick to my stomach. I couldn't breathe - the pressure on my chest was horrendous.

I thought I was having a heart attack. I called for help! Many skilled hands were there almost instantly, covering me with cold cloths, injecting an antihistamine to my IV. The on-call doctor was there directing the ministrations. Finally, after two EpiPen injections into my thigh, the symptoms started to calm down. My oncologist was there as well. Wow, they had called him too. That was scary. I was one of the minority who had a full-blown allergic reaction to this drug. The chemo was stopped for the day and rescheduled for the next week. The offending drug was discontinued. Once I got home, I slept for the rest of the day.

Thoughts during the next week were all over the place. It was tough to get ready and to get into the mindset to go back. Some weeks, as I started to feel better, and the previous chemo was in the rearview mirror, I would be able to go back without a second thought. This time, after the anaphylaxis, I had these thoughts that said, *No way! I can't go back there. Why am I bothering with this? Maybe I should give up and let cancer take over?* Yes, there were times when it got very dark in my mind and spirit. Then, once again, my deep-seated optimism and faith would come to my rescue.

My heartfelt gratitude for all the life lessons I had already experienced began to resurface in my spirit. I had decided to have this chemo as a way to get rid of this cancer. The plan was clear; the paradigm, familiar and straightforward. I needed to deal with it by using the ideas and practices that had come from a lifetime of input into my subconscious. I would not give up when the going was hard. I would not give in to despair or discouragement. My past experiences had shown me that I was on a learning path. All of these experiences had been molding me into the person I was meant to be – fulfilling my life purpose. It was clear to me now that I was here to heal and to teach. These were the thoughts I needed to cultivate if I was to make it through this ordeal. I tried not to allow the darkness in, but it could slip by even the most vigilant mind. The trick here was to get the negative thoughts stopped as quickly as possible and reintroduce the positive outlook that I needed. Remembering that thoughts are things helped me corral the ones that needed to be ousted and bring in constructive ones to visualize the best outcome. Sometimes I used the idea of a basketful of small boards with positive words painted on them. Sunshine lined the bottom of the basket, and all these encouraging words were sitting there, ready to be gathered up by me.

I am convinced that this journey prepared me and gave me experiences to share once I was through this nasty stuff. Oh my! I was so grateful that I was a positive, joyful person way down inside my spirit because I needed that person now. The lesson here is that if you are not naturally a positive person, now is the time to begin. One useful exercise is finding gratitude in every day. To reinforce this habit, I started a Gratitude Journal. The suggested formula to get the most benefit is to write three things that you are grateful for every night. Some nights writing three things that I was thankful for was hard. I would put something like, "I am alive." Or "I am going to sleep, and I can forget the pain and ickiness for a few hours." These may seem to be simple and not significant to you, but believe me when I say there will be days when you need to find even the smallest glimmer of hope to get you through.

The sixth treatment went well, and I was now at the halfway mark. This roller coaster ride was not fun – I would get to feeling okay by the tenth-day post-treatment, only to realize I have to go back for another onslaught a few days later. Physically, the chemo's side effects seemed to be cumulative, meaning it got worse with each episode. The sensation that my hands and feet were filled with needles and pins was just plain annoying. My fingernails were peeling and breaking at every angle. The sores in my mouth made eating very difficult, and food tasted tinny all the time. Even the most minor physical symptoms contributed to a feeling of apprehension. These thoughts would run through my head. *Are the drugs working? Yes, yes, yes! I hope so. I believe so.* Then some anger would surface: *They better be, because this is no picnic.*

I needed to capture that sure knowledge that this was going to come out okay. I always have had trouble understanding one particular scripture, Hebrews 11:1. It states, "Faith is the assured expectation of things hoped for, the evident demonstration of realities though not beheld." Now I found myself leaning into this passage in a whole new way. I held onto the faith that I would be cancer-free in February when they did the first CT scan. I was holding on to the assured expectation that this was working. The next three months would be living that verse of scripture. Stay believing with me.

CHAPTER SIX

Continuing On

*T*he next treatments followed the same routine. It was now commonplace to check-in, have the blood work, get the oncologist's okay, then start the infusion. My body had maintained a healthy platelet count. I'd never had the disappointment of getting the blood tests, only to find out that there was some low count that would make the therapy detrimental, and then having to go home until I was stronger. I think it would have been hard to work around that feeling. It was hard enough to prepare mentally for the scheduled time, let alone having to wait for an improvement in the numbers. I was given the strength to continue, even on the Fridays that going to the Clinic felt like driving to a torture chamber.

The staff was always warm and welcoming. They were kind and supportive. And efficient. There was a no-nonsense attitude there. Yes, this was a grueling process, but the medical staff made it as straight-forward and as painless as possible. Yet as I got into treatments 8 and 9, it took everything I had to go there with a smile and a positive attitude. When I left after several hours with my fanny pack pump delivering more chemo, I imagined each pump pushed healing into those nasty cells. Again, I envisioned that like PacMan, little yellow circles were going after the cancer cells and eating them up. Chomp chomp chomp.

By January, and looking at my last treatment, new thoughts came to torment me. Will I ever get back to normal? When will things taste right, and when will my mouth be healed inside, and the corners of my lips not split? When will there be no blisters and cracks on my fingers? When? Please? When? On nights when I had a good sleep, I woke up hoping that I would have some energy that day. Guess what? Most of the time for the past six months, it has been nope, nada, nyet, none, zero, no energy. Okay, I'm ranting here, but grrrr, I had had enough! One more treatment left! Yay. Then the flip side, a CT scan in February would see what's what... and then?? Positive energy needed! Not to mention the fact that I had been finding it hard to stay up those last few weeks because the fatigue was so debilitating.

Then I get a big boost and a bright ray of sunshine. My daughter came from two thousand miles away to be with me for this last trip to the clinic. I was thrilled. Her visit was the treat that I needed to get through this final week. We went to the clinic together, and she spent the day at my side. We have always been comfortable just sitting in quiet and silence together, and now her presence was a balm to my hurting psyche. I highly recommend finding something which is a delightful treat for your final few weeks of treatment, especially that last one. Her visit was such a gift to me and perhaps to her as well. She finally was able to see where I had all these infusions, meet my medical staff, and learn what I have experienced for the past six months. We are people watchers and love to make up funny scenarios about everyone we see, and even at the cancer clinic, we were able to amuse ourselves with this fun pastime. The visit passed in a flash, and all too soon, Michelle had to go back home to her own life.

Being done with chemo felt like summer vacation. Remember how the end of the school year loomed with final exams and saying goodbye to some friends you wouldn't see for a few months? Now was that time for me, and I was left feeling strangely unoccupied. There was no scheduled appointment in two weeks. I was free!! All that was left was the CT scan, slated for the next month, February. This scan was to check and see what had happened to the cancer over these six months of drug therapy. The results would be a baseline for the periodic checkups over the next year. I was anxious to have this test to have some evidence of my progress.

Again, the hospital staff was the model of efficiency, and before I knew it, the scan was over, and I was out and heading home. The appointment with the doctor was the following week. Many days I still felt tired and sick, but hopeful as well. This whole regimen had worked, hadn't it?

You know what it's like, wanting to hear the news but not wanting to hear it. I was scared to find out in case it was not good. Dave came with me to this critical appointment, his first time to go through the whole routine. I went to the check-in area, had the blood draw, distributed my thank you cards and candies, and then went over to the doctor's office to wait. And wait. The half-hour stretched to an hour. Waiting and waiting. Dave was more than nervous. It hit him that there were some very sick people here, and I had been there for six months along with them.

Finally, my doctor came in. My eyes were glued to him, daring to hope as he checked his computer. Suddenly, his face split into a huge smile, giving away the GGGRRREEEAAATTT news. Nothing showing or suspicious in the scans. Blood work typical. YES! No cancer cells are growing! Hooray! I can't even begin to tell you how good this felt.

Oh, the sigh of relief and feeling of excitement in my heart. I was okay. The chemo had worked. No cancer was growing in my body. *Oh my! Thank you for the continuous prayers, support, and positive thoughts of a big community around me.*

Now I was genuinely free until June, when I would go for a colonoscopy, followed next February, the one-year point, by a CT scan. In the meantime, there would be blood tests to check a cancer marker every month, which was helpful but not definitive enough to be sure that the chemo had completely done its job. I now needed to hang onto the faith that what I had been going through worked. And to trust the doctors and researchers that this was the correct treatment that would give me the best chance to live a long and full life, at least until I'm ninety.

June found me still very, very well. Hooray! Sometimes I couldn't say it enough!! My colonoscopy was one hundred percent clear, right down to the internal incision where the cancer had been. This year had been a tremendous journey. The next question was, "How do I learn to live fully with no cancer?"

I petitioned my doctor to have the port removed. He was reluctant because it was there if we needed it again. I pleaded with him. All my blood tests had been routine, and, in my mind, I don't need that port anymore. He said, "It's fully healed and isn't giving you any trouble. Why not leave it there?" I explained that it bothered me mentally. Every time I showered or wore a low-cut top, I saw and felt it. I wanted this constant reminder of the disease and treatment gone. Finally, the patient prevailed, and the port was removed. This surgery was minor but significant to me. Wow! What an unbelievable boost for me to have it gone! Just a small scar there now.

I continued to feel better each day. It was strange, because some days I thought, *Wow! I CAN do ordinary things now!* One year ago, I was enduring the every-other-week chemo, and it was dragging my energy way down. Now I had regained a lot of energy! I could vacuum the living room, a tiny space, in one shot. I could go shopping without stopping every fifteen minutes to rest. I knew angels and archangels, which I had been studying more and more during this time, played a big part in my renewed health and vitality. I had learned that these amazing creatures are here to help us with everything that we do, and I had been working on allowing them to guide me each day. I was so blessed to have heavenly support! They await our permission to help because, as humans, we are granted free will. The angels must respect that and can only help when we allow them in. Now that I was doing so, life was better than ever, and I was in love with it!

I am well. This reality is difficult to believe. After more than a year of living with the idea that I had cancer, this is a fresh and exciting possibility.

My life is a whole lot better. The mental adjustment to being well is a bit more complicated. Although I tried very hard not to doubt that I would get past cancer, there were times when my mind would go to that other outcome. What if? What if I was going to die soon? What if my life took a detour off the main thought pattern for a while? And what if I couldn't get back on the positive road again?

At this point, I have lived with chronic pain and various symptoms of CFS/fibromyalgia for more than

30 years. This illness is there, but it's not life-threatening in the way that cancer is. I refuse to be defined by any disease, yet I recognize my life and world had centered around cancer, its treatments, and the unknown for the past twelve-plus months. At that moment, I was sure there was no active cancer in my body. But the reality also was that it had been there and could have had a different outcome. We all know people whose bodies have been overcome by disease, despite their best efforts to fight it. I was teetering back and forth. I was indeed well; then again, cancer could still be there - just hiding. I reminded myself again: I can do more and more each day in the week. Yes! I am well.

Once the treatments are over, it is so long, goodbye, take care of yourself, see you next year. I was now on my own without doctors and nurses to remind me of what I needed to be doing. It may sound strange, but the sense of abandonment is sharp. Some of the things they don't tell you initially are the lingering effects of the treatment. In my case, removing ten to twelve inches of the ascending colon means that I will most likely have diarrhea for the rest of my life. First, we tried four anti-diarrhea pills a day to control it, then gradually found a balance at two daily. It's a small concession to make for having the rest of my life. I began to find a new rhythm for my day-to-day activities. I could do most things, though sometimes a little slower than others.

I had just discovered Reiki the month before this whole cancer adventure began. I witnessed the healing power of this energy while in the hospital after surgery. I had been attuned to this energy at Level 1 before starting the treatments. The idea was that I could begin to pull this energy in to help me heal. Yes, I did some of that, but honestly, it wasn't a big part of my spiritual routine. Now I had the time and desire to look into this modality more fully. Was I ready to look at this "woo-woo" side of me? The Reiki energy that I have been experiencing was fantastic.

Reiki is incredibly unique energy from God/Spirit/Universe. It is not my energy or power. It is my being used as a conduit to channel specific energy through me. A trained practitioner can direct this energy toward others. We all have experienced the electricity that gives us a jolt when the air is arid, especially in the winter here up north. We are energy put together in a certain way. Remember your high school physics? I remember learning with a healthy dose of skepticism that the desk I was sitting on in class was just energy in a specific pattern. Now I am using that energy, not like a weird snake oil salesman, but as a spiritual energy healer. Spiritual healing can lead to physical healing. This is a truth that is sometimes misunderstood. Our bodies and minds are totally and completely connected. I find some new teachers in my search for higher spiritual understanding and growth, affirming the body-mind connection. I also begin to journal daily. I finally feel as though I am getting this lesson.

I also took more steps to fulfill the greater purpose I had recently become more aware of, and in this year "off," I qualified as a certified Reiki II Practitioner and started to find clients. I was excited about using this amazing unique energy to continue to support my healing and share it with others. I rented a room at a treatment center on an as-needed basis; I began to work with the YMCA as a Reiki practitioner – they would make the appointments, and I would show up to meet and work with those clients. This new me was very different from the old version. That Marion was unsure and afraid of embracing the spiritual energy around us. Even though I had always felt there was more to this world than the physical elements, I held back at openly discussing this and certainly kept quiet about any deja vu feeling that I did have. The cancer experience has freed me to bask in the light and love from the spiritual realm. We are now at Marion 2.0.

When I heard about the Warrior Walk sponsored by the cancer clinic I attended, I immediately knew I wanted to do it. I had never before walked, run, or jogged at an organized event, yet this was something I felt compelled to do. I practiced walking on my treadmill at home and felt confident that I could make the shorter version of 1 K. Walking, not running for sure. That day the weather was beautiful – sunny with a gentle breeze, and a friend had signed on to walk with me. I was so excited when we got to the designated gathering place and picked up our shirt badges and headscarves with the name and date emblazoned on them. The runners who are doing the 10K distance start first. There was a buzz in the air. The energy was contagious.

Next, the group doing the 5K left the start line, while our smaller group waited for the "Ready. Set. Go." command. When it did, we set off walking a well-used path near the Erie Canal. The sun was beating down on me, and I began to feel the heat. Everyone passed my friend and me, but it was okay. I was not doing this to place in any order, just to do it. The path wound across the Canal, and before we knew it, we were on the home stretch. There was a small shortcut back to the finish line, and considering that I was boiling from the heat and feeling the distance, we took the "out." I did not feel disappointed or like a failure for not entirely completing the full race distance. The important thing was that I had started, did the best I could, and finished! We enjoyed the light lunch the organizers had provided, drank a few bottles of water. I had a winner's attitude and a certificate saying I had participated in a Warrior Walk. Yay.

I do not believe that one can walk with cancer and treatment without some profound changes happening. As a young Reiki client expressed to me, "My friends just don't get it." To survive is to have changed many attitudes, thinking patterns, and basic practices that others take for granted. I was getting the feeling back in my hands and feet, the brain fog that had lingered for so long had begun to dissipate, and I was regaining my sense of taste. All these are happening so slowly that at first, I didn't recognize the progress. Wait, did that just taste like chocolate pudding? Whoo, I began to trust it. Yes, I still needed a nap every so often, but the overwhelming fatigue started to lift.

One of the most insightful revelations from the angels is to refer to the cancer as "the" cancer rather than owning it and saying *my* cancer. This small adjustment has had an intense impact on me. I don't want ownership of that disease. The difference between *the* and *my* is vast. Think about this! Our language, the words that we use out loud, and how we talk to ourselves inside our heads matter. Be mindful of those subtle ideas that sneak into your thoughts. Think about it: is it easier to get rid of something that you refer to as *the item* or as *my item*?

Let's face it. I was a completely different person after the disease and treatment. The "before" me was drifting along, working, and anticipating semi-retirement. I had abandoned most of the mindful practices of my earlier life and was basically in a rut. We had an online tire business that had been very successful but had begun to dwindle in the last year. We officially closed that door, and I had a lot more spare time to whittle away with busy work. Dealing with the active treatment had filled the past few years. Now it was time to examine where I was. The physical side of the situation was challenging, certainly. Coping with that side bothered Dave the most. For me, the mental side was far more troublesome. I needed to switch my thoughts back from being in the attack mode to being in the living mode. While actively fighting cancer, our minds are filled with those day-to-day battles. Once we're done with these actions and mental preparation, we must now figure out how to live again without the constant focus on the fight. This is not a straight-forward transition. There were many times during this transition when I needed to go back and read, again and again, the words of encouragement, the sweet thoughts in the many get-well cards and when I need-ed friends and family in my corner. I was, and still am, truly grateful that so many were here with me on this difficult and scary journey through hell from which I was now emerging.

CHAPTER SEVEN

One Year Later

❦

*I*t had been one year since the CT scan that had served as a baseline for future assessment. As I headed for my first annual checkup, I felt like I was about to take a major final exam I had been working towards for the whole year. Had I worked hard enough at keeping the cancer at bay? Had I done everything I needed to do? During the months of diagnosis, surgery, and treatment, it was easier to keep my mind on the activities and mindset required for that battle.

I arrived hopeful, yet fearful. This scan and check-up were a big deal. Having the scan is easy – it's the waiting to get the results that is complicated. I want the news but am terrified that it will be awful. And, indeed, a few days later, I learned it was NOT good news. Like the Terminator, it was back! There was a swollen lymph node near my navel that could be cancer. The doctors needed a biopsy to be sure before we could discuss any treatment. The first attempt at getting tissue samples was not successful, as this node was in a very inaccessible place. We started seeing various technicians and specialists who try to get a biopsy. The seemingly last resort was a doctor who is fondly known as the "Biopsy Whisperer." He scheduleed an active CT scan and was in charge of a long and flexible needle. As he watched the screen, he carefully guided the probe delicately through the organs and other assorted "stuff," and finally, with a cry of victory, reached the offending node and clipped some tissue samples to be tested.

After all this drama, it was almost anticlimactic to find there is a new active cancer in this lymph node. The sense of failure and dread overtook me for a few minutes. This message was not what I wanted to hear.

Once again, my past training and learning began to bubble up inside. Okay, cancer had metastasized to a new place. What do we do to get rid of it? It was somewhat comforting to be scheduling another port install, booking the chemo treatments. Bizarrely I fell into the routine quickly; in fact, it was almost a relief to have something concrete to do. The whole year in between had been ethereal, fuzzy, and with no definite landmarks to show that this crazy cancer was still there growing inside of me. Going for the blood test, having the chemo infusion, and the weekend pump are familiar. I realized now that my inner self had been craving those tests and those outward signs. Now that is sick! (I mean, mentally ill.) I knew that I needed help. I sought out spiritual teachers and read and studied more about the effects of the mind on the body. I could see that I had not learned the lesson thoroughly. The Universe and the angels were giving me another round of learning and another chance at figuring out what was next on my path.

The drug regime was changed to try and get rid of every active cancer cell in my body. Did it feel different? Well, yes and no. There was a sense of déjà vu. I had been here before, but I had begun to change my mental attitude in the year off. Changing your thinking is crucial to this journey. *Can I survive this again? Am I living each day mindful and grateful?* Often, we look far ahead and think I'll do that when – "when I am thin," "when I am rich," or "when I am healthy." But no! The message is clear. Today is *it*. We cannot wait until something else happens. This truth hit me in a big way. We only have now. Am I living my day my life today to its fullest, or have I been drifting again?

I made a new friend who insisted on coming with me to the cancer clinic each time. She was younger and interested in helping me to cope. I agreed that she could be with me, and found a different experience having someone right there. I often slept through the whole treatment, too tired to be concerned about my friend's time. This experience was another lesson for me. I learned that I needed to put my needs first right now and spend all my energy on getting better. With my role as a lifelong caretaker, this was a hard lesson for me to absorb.

A friend invited me to try a labyrinth walk. What is this? I googled it to find out that a labyrinth is an ancient geometric pattern that, over hundreds of years, has become a place for meditating, and a spiritual place for soothing and bringing clarity into one's life. I began to walk on it regularly and invited a few supportive friends to come along the evening before each scheduled treatment. I found it a relaxing and spiritual time to prepare me mentally for the next procedure.

After a month or two of the chemo, I noticed redness and oozing around my port, more severe nausea, and generally feeling more lousy than usual. I delayed the next chemo treatment because of how sick I was. I was at the Emergency Department two weekends in a row with nothing definite diagnosed. The third weekend was the breaking point for me. I was vomiting and hot and feverish, and in such agony, with pain in my abdomen, I could not stand it. I called the home care nurse, and he came to check me out. His recommendation was to go to the hospital immediately. It was nearly 10:00 pm on Saturday, and I am reluctant to go because I am thinking about the long lines on the weekend at the Emergency Department. But the pain and sickness prevail, so I went. When the triage nurse noted my symptoms and the fact that I was a cancer patient, she bumped me up on the intake list.

After that, there was only a short wait before they ushered me into the unit, then to a private, separate room. My temperature spiked; my blood pressure was out of control. The team tried everything to figure out what was going on, but they did not know what was causing this severe distress to my body. They drew blood and took swabs from near the port, then wheeled me out to get a CT scan of my lower abdomen. By this time, I was nearly delirious with pain. The severity of the situation hit me when the doctor asked if I had a DNR in place. Whoa! Am I dying? I called on my angelic support team to help me through this, and I pray for answers before it is too late. Finally, the tests showed a staph infection in my port and a twisted bowel obstruction in my lower abdomen. Neither was related to the cancer or the treatments. I was placed in quarantine, with extreme cautionary measures in place. Saturday turns into an exceptionally long night.

Sometime before morning, I was transferred to a private room in the cancer clinic — what a pure luxury. Everyone who worked there, from doctors to the cleaning staff and even the sweet people who bring in food, were all aware that I was in the midst of chemo-therapy and had a compromised immune system. They all wore protective gowns, masks, and gloves, which were stripped off at the door and deposited in a special laundry basket.

The next day my daughter and her fiancé flew in from thousands of miles away. I was delighted to see them. My daughter and I have always had a special bond. They came up every day to spend the time with me. I was so incredibly sick that I just acknowledged their presence, thankful when they got me water, and helped make me comfortable. It was ten days of hell, and also a very bizarre time. My body is still under attack. Questions flood my mind. What am I doing wrong? Why is this happening? And how much more can I take? As I slowly got better, I realized that amidst the pain and misery, I had been in a time of intense soul-searching.

The doctor decided to remove the port, which would be the best way to treat the infection. Finally, the twisted bowel resolved itself, and I was relieved of that pain. The staph infection would take a lot longer to clear up. There was a short procedure to insert a PICC line in my arm, and I was well enough to find this fascinating. It was done by a very specialized and skilled nurse practitioner. The attendant took me on this long ride, down corridors, around many corners, and past all sorts of interesting rooms to a lab that seemed miles from my hospital room. I remember hoping he could find our way back! Again, a glimmer of gratitude slipped in.

We were on a track to recovery for this set of side ailments. The next day I was sent home with antibiotics — a daily injection that I would administer myself, with the vials of medication that the Home Care Service would deliver to my door. I was feeling better and thought I could handle this for thirty days. There would be no chemo for a while, and we would decide what happened after all the acute infections cleared up. My daughter took me to the clinic for a check-in with my doctor. I was too weak to walk, so she had to push me in a wheelchair. As much as this bothered me and made me feel very ill, I was sure that it was absolutely devastating for her. She hadn't been around me for the months of this disease, so suddenly, seeing her mother in such a vulnerable state must have been one of the toughest times for her. Sometimes in our world of illness, we don't notice the destructive effect on our loved ones. I was grateful that she was with me, and I tried to remember her perspective as she willingly pushed me around!

This past month had been the most frightening time of the past almost two years. I had spent that year "off" from cancer and chemotherapy, trying to restart my life. The news that the colon cancer had *metastasized* to a new place – the significant health ordeal that followed – was a catastrophic experience that further catapulted me into changing my thinking and my life.

Cancer was the beginning of that for me, and that near-death experience due to the staph infection and bowel obstruction combo marked me in a profound way. I needed to get serious about what I was doing and start living mindfully. I began meditating in earnest. I connected with the angels, archangels, and other Ascended Masters. I realized that before I could step more fully into my role as healer and teacher, I needed to first mentally and physically heal me.

The CT scan in June showed the cancer was still in the lymph node and the three months of chemo before the severe illness had not cleared any of it. The oncologist was reluctant to continue with chemo and preferred to go to radiation. After much thought, I opted to stay with the familiar for a while. I wanted to keep with the current regimen and finish the other three months of chemotherapy. To do this involved having another port installed on the opposite side of my chest. I needed to wait until the "staph" doctor clears me before this could happen – a reasonable precaution as I do not want that infection to transfer to the new port!

In August, the end of the six months of the scheduled chemotherapy, another CT scan shows the same pesky lymph node hanging on to those nasty cells. This time, no more chemo was ordered. I now felt as though I knew some of the angels in my world. I accepted that they were with me to heal and continue to grow in my service to God/Spirit. I talked with a spiritual advisor, and we decided to involve visualization and work with the archangels. Each day I visualized Archangel Michael taking his sword and cutting out the cancer cells. I then invoked Archangel Raphael pouring his soothing green light in filling it with a healing balm. By the September CT scan, no cancer was showing in that node!! The cancer clinic had advocated visualization, meditation, and it was working! Suddenly, I was once again back on track to living a "normal" life. A PET scan was scheduled for December; for now, my daily spiritual routine focuses mainly on meditation and journaling.

CHAPTER EIGHT

Radiation Rocks

That December, they discovered a newly-infected lymph node in my abdomen, shining brightly on the PET scan. Radiation was the recommended treatment because the chemo had ravaged my entire body to the point that more chemo could be more detrimental than the cancer itself. Just how much the chemo has affected me was astonishing. They now needed a special light to find the veins in my arms to draw blood. This machine was fascinating. I watched with wonder and awe as the bluish bulb highlights the weird roadmap my veins had become. Who knew? My once very ordinary veins now were jagged odd pathways. No part of me had not suffered from the onslaught of the poison used to kill the cancer cells. I am so grateful that at least the chemo part was over, for now. The advancements in radiation have made this treatment less invasive than it was even five years earlier. Radiation is also a significant attack on the cancer cells, but it is pinpointed and limited to the area where it is needed. I met a new team of oncologists whose specialty is in radiation therapy, then reported to the radiation clinic for the initial mapping and establishing of the area to be radiated.

The way that they accomplished this exact action was also fascinating. I laid on an x-ray table on top of a body-length beanbag. Using a scan, they pinpointed the spots and angles that the laser rays needed to hit and bounce off to target that one lymph node. I was settled into the exact position so that the radiation machine could send its rays to the pesky cancer located near my belly button. The technicians pushed all the beans around my body so that every curve and bump was included. Next, they sucked all the air out of the bag until the soft bean bag became a sturdy, firm mold of me. I felt like a giant chocolate Easter Bunny, molded-in so nicely. I was tattooed with dots in several locations to ensure that the radiation beams went where they needed to. *How cool is this? My first tattoos!* I was amazed at the ingenuity and brilliance of the minds that developed this system. I would have seven treatments, five in one week and two the next.

When it was time for a radiation treatment, my mold was placed on the table. I climbed up and settled into the exact position needed. The staff then set little lead nuggets on the tattooed dots. The machine moved over and around me in an arc. The beams hit each marker and bounced on to the cancer node like I was in a giant pinball machine. This action attacked the cancerous node from all sides. Astounding! The whole process took only minutes. When the bells and whistles stopped, I got up and out of the mold, whole and no, *not* made of chocolate.

The main side effect was exhaustion. Before having radiation, I thought I knew what being tired was. After all, I am no stranger to weariness. I'd had CFS for more than thirty-five years, not to mention the chemo. But this was a whole new feeling of bone-deep, incapacitating tiredness. I spent the next few hours napping, sleeping, resting, and then the next day doing it all over again. The exhaustion would persist for several months. Although the treatments had been completed, this lingering side effect made it difficult to get going with my "normal" life again.

After the radiation treatments, I had to wait three months before getting another PET scan. As this day approached, I was filled with emotions and questions. Am I done? I'd thought I was done with this disease two years ago. Then, whoops, think again. What happened? Have I finally learned the lessons I needed to know during these three years of dealing with the big C? I believe that everything in life happens to teach us something, some improvement, or attitude adjustment that we need to live out our purpose — attitudes like patience, joy, empathy. I have discerned my purpose here on earth — to teach and to heal. Accomplishing and working on my path begins with me. I am the number one project. All of this is to teach me something. What is it? Or was it many things I had begun to review over the past three years? What had I learned? "I am loved," is the answer that comes to me quickly.

Right here at home, Dave had shown this love over and over. Assembling meals, doing the dishes, things that he'd never had to do in his entire life. All around me, family and friends showered me with food, cards, loving words, and more. Friends dropped by for a quick visit, bringing me a laugh or two, hugs, and love. Again, and again, these actions taught me how to be a receiver. I was usually the giver, so this was a challenging lesson for me. This lesson was necessary for two reasons. First, I needed to be humble and recognize just how much I needed to accept these loving actions. Second, and even more critical in my role as teacher and healer, I needed to provide open space for others to give and grow. These actions encompassed both branches of my life purpose. I was teaching and healing at the same time. Healing is both physical and spiritual. Always being the giver is selfish. It is haughty. It is prideful. Not in the sense of "look at me, I am so great," but in the spirit, saying, "I am not worthy and do not need your giving. I can do this on my own. I am a dependable one here." Can you see how not accepting and allowing these loving actions and expressions will stifle the others' growth?

Those months waiting for a clean PET scan were filled with more soul searching. Does this sound repetitive? It seemed so for me. I thought that I had figured out what was going on in my life and what I would be doing for the rest of it way back two years ago when I finished the chemotherapy and all that. But I just couldn't get the hang of it, nor the mental attitude to get on with it. Do you know what I mean? Maybe you have planned on getting right back to your "normal" life but found that it wasn't that easy to do. You get up with a plan one day, but that old exhaustion comes and knocks you for a loop. And motivation flies right out the window. It's okay! It is what happens when your body is under attack from cancer first, then the treatments of either chemotherapy, radiation, or both. Now there I was again, another year filled with concern and working on physical healing. I look back at the last three years. Year one: diagnosis, surgery, chemotherapy. Year two: one CT scan, one colonoscopy, and then bye, bye, little contact with the cancer clinic or anyone connected to it in any way. Year three: more cancer, more chemotherapy, radiation, many more physical issues, some related to the therapy, some just run of the mill illness from ordinary living with a severely damaged body, ending with a PET scan.

I want to assure you that this time hasn't been all spent on dealing with the crappy cancer and its ill effects. In waiting for what I hope to be my first ever clean PET scan, I completed the required training and became a Reiki Master. This step is significant in my spiritual growth. Being a Master means that I now have a more direct connection to this energy. The angels are around me and accessible with this energy. I am qualified to teach and attune others to Reiki as well. Such a privilege! Reiki helps with my mental attitude as well as helping me with physical issues. As I was once again in wait-and-see mode, I began overseeing the renovation of the front part of our house to use as a wellness center. Dave and I live in an old farmhouse that had extensions added on over the years. We have used the front two rooms to store vintage furniture from my husband's grandmother's home. We have not used it as a living space for years. Now - aha! - I realized it was the perfect place for my business. These rooms also have the advantage of being rent-free. Do you get this little concession? I seemed to be building in a safety valve if I had to take the time to recover. As I waited for the scan results, I opened Chrysalis Wellness Center, a place for teaching and healing body, mind, and spirit.

Finally, the day came for the appointment with the oncologist. Dave accompanied me on this trip. We are both nervous and worried, but I put on a happy face, and away we go.

CHAPTER NINE

Follow Up

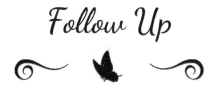

The three years of the rollercoaster ride of *Yes, it's there; now maybe it's not; oh wait, yes, there is some more*, was finally over. The scans were clear. Oh, there was a funny-looking lymph node still there, but it was not lighting up with any activity. The verdict was that I had no active cancer in my body. Let me repeat this. No cancer. None. Nada. Zero. Relief poured over me. We had done it. This was the time. In the past, the feeling and news that we'd heard conveyed were a wait and see approach. The doctors said things like: "We think that we got all the cancer cells, but we are keeping a close eye on everything." The scans were to check on this progress. Three times there was something there to treat. Now, for the first time, the scan was *clear*. Tears of joy filled my eyes.

My husband let out a massive sigh of relief. This uncertainty of the past three years had been hard on him too. I quickly texted my family and close friends. The question most people asked was, "Are you sure?" Part of me wanted to answer, "Yes! I can go on living. I can go to work." The other part of me said, "Don't ask!"

I wanted to get on with my life, but how to do this? We think that we have finished with this ongoing battle against the hideous disease of cancer. I had put all my energy into this fight. I am trying to believe the words, "Yes, this is finally finished." But thoughts sneak in. *I've heard that before. Yeah, right, we've been down this road before.* Once again, the work on *Me* intensifies.

I am not a routine type of person. I prefer to be spontaneous. When I was young, I remember getting married and defining what kind of life I would have as a woman responsible for the household. I was determined to make spontaneity a priority for me. Influenced by the TV sit-coms of the time, I decided never to have such a tight routine that we did the laundry on Monday and eat meatloaf every Tuesday. I am a somewhat organized person and love to be in control, and oh, I love lists, To-Do lists, food plan lists for the week, but my schedule would be filled with a variety of different chores and different meals on different days. I am telling you this because having a routine is highly recommended by personal growth and spiritual gurus. Every book I pick up, every blog post I read, say the same thing. A mindful routine is vital to developing a powerful spiritual self. Remember Maxwell Maltz's examples of how we create the habit of thinking positively? Repetition and even rituals help to establish practices. I know for sure that I must continue exploring every avenue for healing and living a healthy life. I need to get past this hang-up and learn to live with structure. That takes discipline, and unfortunately, a routine is one of the best ways to establish that discipline.

Plans, ideas, and activities started flying through my mind. Restarting my life was exciting. What would I do first? Scrambling around, I found that I was doing bits of this and that. I needed to get a handle on this new enormous concept now that I had a life again. What did I need to do first? Of course, I began by making a list. I designed a daily routine with times and estimated completion goals. Meditation would begin each day, at the same time every morning, and journaling right after that. The house would be tidy and clean, given my new schedule. I had days for working, days, and times for playing, for cleaning. I got a thrill just by looking at my daily bullet journal with all the details listed. Then reality reared its chaotic head! I would sleep in and miss the scheduled meditation time. The day devolved into a feeling yucky, tired kind of day. The schedule had lasted about four days! Now what? How do I restart? For more than three years, my life has been defined by tests, scans, treatments, anticipation of and preparation for therapies, and worry. I say again, now what?

We have all been there, haven't we? When plans are made, and then they get screwed up because of circumstances. I realize that it is going to take more than a list to keep me motivated. I feel a sense of disappointment. I am hard on ME. Things like "you've been through all this rough stuff in the past three years and know that you have things to do, yet here you are, doing nothing!" I stop. I catch myself quickly. What have I learned? Yes! I can get right back on track and accomplish meaningful things. I remember that I was able to complete the commitment to myself to get through the chemo, the radiation, and the physical deterioration of parts of my body. I sit quietly, meditating, and ask the angels to help me show up for myself once again. I am encouraged by the feelings I experience. The thoughts that pop into my mind are positive reinforcement. It's okay to fall or miss a few days on the schedule. I forgive myself and start again. There is an 80/20 rule that governs successful people. This rule says that as long as you are on track eighty percent of the time and allow for detours the other twenty percent, things will work out for you. So, day four was part of the twenty percent off-course time. By day six, I was back on track.

The next year was a mix of two steps forward and one step back. Mentally I wasn't quite ready to believe that I had survived. The "why me?" thought popped in, which I found intriguing. I didn't have that idea or ask that question about getting cancer, but now I am asking, "Why have I survived?" I was then reminded of my purpose again: to teach and to heal. The future is and always would be now, and it begins right here with me. I need to love myself, forgive myself, and to live in gratitude and joy.

CHAPTER TEN

Re-entering the Real World

*T*he next scan three months later was also clear, and so was the one three months following that. Even the oncologist was smiling now. It appears cancer, like Elvis, had left the building. I was beginning to trust this. I have now graduated to having a scan in six months! This time frame may not seem to be much of a victory, but oh, this news feels so good. I was now entering the end of the first year of clean scans. I loved this idea.

On the negative side, there were still some prolonged effects of cancer and treatments. Not all of these were physical. Mentally there were lots of hurdles to overcome. One consequence that is widespread in the cancer survivor community is what is known as Chemo Brain. This is real, and it is annoying. The brain fog that came during the actual treatments was still a part of my daily life. I had experienced this effect from the Chronic Fatigue Syndrome for the past thirty years, and now it is compounded by the chemotherapy drugs. It appears in those times when the word you are searching for just won't show up, and more frustrating is that it isn't "just on the tip of your tongue." No, it has gone, gone into a black hole in your brain.

The good news is that we can overcome some of this with the application of remarkable techniques being taught and used by holistic healers and medical personnel in various hospitals around the USA. Other scientific research shows that we can heal the damage done to our cells with other holistic techniques.

The approach developed by Dr. Joe Dispenza, who has spent decades educating thousands on how they can rewire their brains and bring their bodies in line with those changes. (There is a link to his website and YouTube channel in the appendix.) Do you know that meditation can retrain your neurotransmitters to find new connections and create new pathways to overcome some of that brain disruption? As Dispenza wrote on May 8, 2020 post of his blog, Inner Mission, " .... the totality of our scientific measurements that prove our mind and will have the power to change biological functions..."

You will be a different person along your journey whether you graduate to being a survivor or you graduate out of this lifetime. The physical stuff happens and just is. The mental and spiritual self is where significant changes occur. This experience changed me, and most certainly changed my husband. He has his own story to tell, yet I will say that he has become calmer, more open-minded, and allowed his sense of humor to re-emerge.

Since reaching that celebrated state of "survivor," I have been searching and looking into anything that offers a spark of hope to keep this monster at bay. I absorbed all that I could about Reiki energy and now use it every day. I started looking into other alternate solutions. I am so grateful that I have a curious mind that craves knowledge. The tough times I faced first in 2014 with discovering cancer growing in me and then the near-death experience I had in 2016 have made me realize just how much I can still learn and how much I can do to help myself and others. My epiphany led me to another energy source of healing called Integrated Energy Therapy. This methodology works with a group of angels who help clear the negative energy stored in our bodies. Often this negative force appears as a disease of some sort or other. You know that tension in the back of your neck that you feel when working at your computer for a long time. A combination of Reiki and IET can help to soften those tight muscles and relieve the tension. IET energy works directly with your body's cellular memory and energy field to get the "issues out of your tissues" for good. IET helps you to release limiting energy patterns safely and gently from your past, empower and balance your life in the present, and embody your full potential as you move into the future. The classes to learn this technique are fun and enlightening. This new modality of healing gives me another arrow in my quiver to use for myself and to help others.

In the past six-plus years, I have learned a lot about

meditation, keeping a great attitude no matter the circumstances, especially by associating with spiritual people, using a daily journal to keep me present, and keeping me organized and growing. I suggest that if you haven't used any of these tools, you look into them and look into other ideas that come to you for you to heal inside and out.

These are some of the ways I have chosen to improve my mental and physical health. Are they right for you? Only you can decide on the steps you need to take to negotiate your path in this new role as a survivor. But you will need to do something different to handle the latest you. The old you had cancer, and although it may reoccur for many of us, you and I are new people. Change does happen. You can do one of two things. Let it happen with little or no input from you or take charge of your life and live purposely and with gratitude.

The God of my understanding can be trusted to send the help, direction, and guidance we need. The angels are messengers waiting to deliver it. All we are required to do is show up and be open to receive it.

Be present. Be here. See everything with wonder and mystery. Face each day with courage, joy, and gratitude. It's worth it.

APPENDIX

Finances

One of the areas I have not yet discussed is the financial burden that cancer and treatments can impose on you and your family. The procedures and scans cost us about $650.00 a month (2014-2017)in co-pays. You can see that over the years, we spent thousands of dollars with extra out-of-pocket expenses. Often this is a burden that the family has a difficult time handling. I am grateful that we were able to cover this. We were able to negotiate a discounted rate with the hospital and clinic when our income dropped, but this dollar figure is the average over that time. Check with a social worker at your hospital or cancer clinic for help with finances.

Planning for Death and Dying

Some essential items to prepare consist of a will, a Power of Attorney, a Healthcare Proxy (called a "Living Will" in some areas), and a DNR (Do Not Resuscitate order). I understand that most of us do not want to do these things or even think about them, but they are vital and necessary for peace of mind for you, your family, or whoever is handling these details.

Taking care of these matters is not a morbid idea but a practical one. Make sure those around you know your wishes in the event of your death or the use of various machines for sustaining life. Think of it as a gift to them, having your specific preferences in writing, and dealing with the practical details sure in the knowledge that it is what you would have wanted. Get this done.

Resources for Cancer Patients and Their Support System

I suggest that you check in your area for these types of agencies:

American Cancer Society

1-800-227-2345

www.cancer.org

Cancer Care, Inc.

1-800-813-4673

www.cancercare.org

Gilda's Clubs

Type this name in your search engine for the one in your area.

Lance Armstrong Foundation

www.livestrong.org

National Cancer Institute

1-800-422-6237

www.cancer.gov

Cancer Connect

Choose the type of cancer in the list for specific information.

https://news.cancerconnect.com/colon-cancer/

https://cancerconnect.com/

People, Places, And Books to Check Out Online

Marion Andrews

www.marionandrews.com

www.chrysaliswellnesscenter.com

Dr. Joe Dispenza

https://drjoedispenza.com/

Becoming Supernatural: How Common People Are Doing the Uncommon

https://marionandrews.com/recommendations/

Breaking The Habit of Being Yourself: How to Lose Your Mind and Create a New One

https://marionandrews.com/recommendations/

Psycho-cybernetics: A new way to get more living out of life

https://marionandrews.com/recommendations/

The Women of Lemuria: Ancient Wisdom for Modern Times

By Monika Muranyi

https://marionandrews.com/recommendations/

Interview with an Angel: An Angel Reveals Astonishing Truths About Life and Death, Religion, the Afterlife, Extraterrestrials, the Power of Love and More

By Stevan J. Thayer

https://marionandrews.com/recommendations/

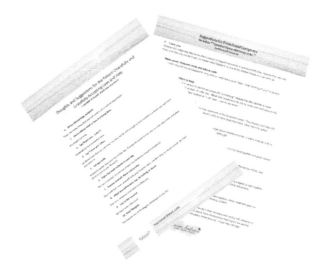

Get Your Free Caregiver's Guide

Often we hold back from being there for them because we don't know what we can say or how we can help. This guide will help you get started.

Get Your Free Patient Guide

This guide includes handy tips to help you through your cancer journey.

Both guides are available on this page, where you can also opt-in for my blog and an occasional newsletter.

www.marionandrews.com/free-guide

ABOUT THE AUTHOR

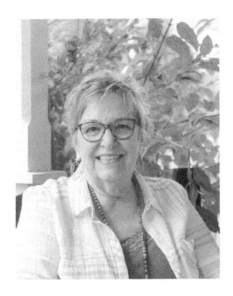

Marion Andrews is an Integrated Energy Therapy Master-Instructor, Reiki Master/Teacher, Life Aficionado, Meditation Coach, bestselling author, and cancer survivor.

Marion has spent the past few years sharing her light and love as she traveled the road with cancer. Following her initial diagnosis with Stage 3B colon cancer, she underwent the recommended chemotherapy, only to repeat the whole scene the following year with the new designation of Stage 4, and then AGAIN the year after that! Told with humor, hope, honesty, and unique insights, her story will take you on a powerful journey that begins with her diagnosis and ends with her being transformed, more vital than ever, and gloriously grateful for all she experienced.

Along with her daughter, Michelle Forsyth, Marion co-authored *Who Am I, Anyway?: A Guided Journal*. She has also contributed to these best-selling books: *111 Morning Meditations; Happy Thoughts Playbook; Healer: 22 Expert Healers Share Their Wisdom to Help You Transform; Kindness Crusader;* and *When I Rise, I Thrive*. All are available on Amazon and through her website at www.marionandrews.com/books

Marion owns Chrysalis Wellness Center, a holistic healing and treatment center located in a farmhouse built in 1847 and decorated with antique furniture from the early 1900s. Marion lives with her husband, Dave, in the remainder of this delightful old house.

You may contact Marion at marion@marionandrews.com or through her website www.marionandrews.com. Subscribe to her blog at www.gloriouslygrateful.com.

Made in United States
North Haven, CT
25 March 2023

34542026R00055